DIET AND WEIGHT LOSS

OLA OBEMBE

This book is dedicated to my family and friends, especially those who sees the value and importance of diets in the process of lossing weight.

Contents

CHAPTER ONE

Eight Best Diet Plans — Sustainability, Weight Loss, and More

It's estimated that nearly half of American adults attempt to lose weight each year. One of the best ways to lose weight is by changing your diet. Yet, the sheer number of available diet plans may make it difficult to get started, as you're unsure which one is most suitable, sustainable, and effective.

Some diets aim to curb your appetite to reduce your food intake, while others suggest restricting your intake of calories and either carbs or fat. What's more, many offer health benefits that go beyond weight loss.

Here are the 8 best diet plans to help you shed weight and improve your overall health.

Share on Pinterest

1. Intermittent fasting

Intermittent fasting is a dietary strategy that cycles between periods of fasting and eating. Various forms exist, including the 16/8 method, which involves limiting your calorie intake to 8 hours per day, and the 5:2 method, which restricts your daily calorie intake to 500–600 calories twice per week.

How it works: Intermittent fasting restricts the time you're allowed to eat, which is a simple way to reduce your calorie intake. This can lead to weight loss — unless you compensate by eating too much food during allowed eating periods.

Weight loss: In a review of studies, intermittent fasting was shown to cause 3–8% weight loss over 3–24 weeks, which is a significantly greater percentage than other methods The same review showed that this way of eating may reduce waist circumference by 4–7%, which is a marker for harmful belly fat

Other studies found that intermittent fasting can increase fat burning while preserving muscle mass, which can improve metabolism

Other benefits: Intermittent fasting has been linked to anti-aging effects, increased insulin sensitivity, improved brain health, reduced inflammation, and many other benefits

Downsides: In general, intermittent fasting is safe for most healthy adults. That said, those sensitive to drops in their blood sugar levels, such as some people with diabetes, low weight, or an eating disorder, as well as pregnant or breastfeeding women, should talk to a health professional before starting intermittent fasting.

Summary Intermittent

fasting cycles between periods of fasting and eating. It has been shown to aid weight loss and is linked to many other health benefits.

2. Plant-based diets

Plant-based diets may help you lose weight. Vegetarianism and veganism are the most popular versions, which restrict animal products for health, ethical, and environmental reasons.

However, more flexible plant-based diets also exist, such as the flexitarian diet, which is a plant-based diet that allows eating animal products in moderation.

How it works: There are many types of vegetarianism, but most involve eliminating all meat, poultry, and fish. Some vegetarians may likewise avoid eggs and dairy.

The vegan diet takes it a step further by restricting all animal products, as well as animal-derived products like dairy, gelatin, honey, whey, casein, and albumin. There are no clear-cut rules for the flexitarian diet, as it's a lifestyle change rather than a diet. It encourages eating mostly fruits, vegetables, legumes, and whole grains but allows for protein and animal products in moderation, making it a popular alternative.

Many of the restricted food groups are high in calories, so limiting them may aid in weight loss.

Weight loss: Research shows that plant-based diets are effective for weight loss. A review of 12 studies including 1,151 participants found that people on a plant-based diet lost an average of 4.4 pounds (2 kg) more than those who included animal products Plus, those following a vegan diet lost an average of 5.5 pounds (2.5 kg) more than people not eating a plant-based diet

Plant-based diets likely aid weight loss because they tend to be rich in fiber, which can help you stay fuller for longer, and low in high-calorie fat

Other benefits: Plant-based diets have been linked to many other benefits, such as a reduced risk of chronic conditions like heart disease, certain cancers, and diabetes. They can also be more environmentally sustainable than meat-based diets

Downsides: Though plant-based diets are healthy, they can restrict important nutrients that are typically found in animal products, such as iron, vitamin B12, vitamin D, calcium, zinc, and omega-3 fatty acids. A flexitarian approach or proper supplementation can help account for these nutrients.

Summary Plant-based diets restrict meat and animal products for various reasons. Studies show that they aid weight loss by reducing your calorie intake and offer many other benefits.

3. Low-carb diets

Low-carb diets are among the most popular diets for weight loss. Examples include the Atkins diet, ketogenic (keto) diet, and low-carb, high-fat (LCHF) diet. Some varieties reduce carbs more drastically than others. For instance, very-low-carb diets like the keto diet restrict this macronutrient to under 10% of total calories, compared with 30% or less for other types

How it works: Low-carb diets restrict your carb intake in favor of protein and fat.

They're typically higher in protein than low-fat diets, which is important, as protein can help curb your appetite, raise your metabolism, and conserve muscle mass In very-low-carb diets like keto, your body begins using fatty acids rather than carbs for energy by converting them into ketones. This process is called ketosis

Weight loss: Many studies indicate that low-carb diets can aid weight loss and may be more effective than conventional low-fat diets. For example, a review of 53 studies including 68,128 participants found that low-carb diets resulted in significantly more weight loss than low-fat diets. What're more, low-carb diets appear to be quite effective at burning harmful belly fat

Other benefits: Research suggests that low-carb diets may reduce risk factors for heart disease, including high cholesterol and blood pressure levels. They may also improve blood sugar and insulin levels in people with type 2 diabetes

Downsides: In some cases, a low-carb diet may raise LDL (bad) cholesterol levels. Very low-carb diets can also be difficult to follow and cause digestive upset in some people. In very rare situations, following a very-low-carb diet may cause a condition known as ketoacidosis, a dangerous metabolic condition that can be fatal if left untreated

Summary Low-carb diets restrict your carb intake, which encourages your body to use more fat as fuel. They can help you lose weight and offer many other benefits.

4. The paleo diet

The paleo diet advocates eating the same foods that your hunter-gatherer ancestors allegedly ate. It's based on the theory that modern diseases are linked to the Western diet, as proponents believe that the human body hasn't evolved to process legumes, grains, and dairy.

How it works: The paleo diet advocates eating whole foods, fruits, vegetables, lean meats, nuts, and seeds. It restricts the consumption of processed foods, grains, sugar, and dairy, though some less restrictive versions allow for some dairy products like cheese.

Weight loss: Numerous studies have shown that the paleo diet can aid weight loss and reduce harmful belly fat

For example, in one 3-week study, 14 healthy adults following a paleo diet lost an average of 5.1 pounds (2.3 kg) and reduced their waist circumference — a marker for belly fat — by an average of 0.6 inches (1.5 cm). Research also suggests that the paleo diet may be more filling than popular diets like the Mediterranean diet and low-fat diets. This may be due to its high protein content

Other benefits: Following the paleo diet may reduce several heart disease risk factors, such as high blood pressure, cholesterol, and triglyceride levels

Downsides: Though the paleo diet is healthy, it restricts several nutritious food groups, including legumes, whole grains, and dairy.

Summary The paleo diet advocates eating whole foods, similar to how your ancestors ate. Studies show that it may aid weight loss and reduce heart disease risk factors.

5. Low-fat diets

Like low-carb diets, low-fat diets have been popular for decades. In general, a low-fat diet involves restricting your fat intake to 30% of your daily calories. Some very- and ultra-low-fat diets aim to limit fat consumption to under 10% of calories

How it works: Low-fat diets restrict fat intake because fat provides about twice the number of calories per gram, compared with the other two macronutrients — protein and carbs. Ultra-low-fat diets contain fewer than 10% of calories from fat, with approximately 80% of calories coming from carbs and 10% from protein. Ultra-low-fat diets are mainly plant-based and limit meat and animal products.

Weight loss: As low-fat diets restrict calorie intake, they can aid in weight loss. An analysis of 33 studies including over 73,500 participants found that following a low-fat diet led to small but relevant changes in weight and waist circumference

However, while low-fat diets appear to be as effective as low-carb diets for weight loss in controlled situations, low-carb diets seem to be the more effective day today

Ultra-low-fat diets are successful, especially among people with obesity. For example, an 8-week study in 56 participants found that eating a diet comprising 7–14% fat led to an average weight loss of 14.8 pounds (6.7 kg)

Other benefits: Low-fat diets have been linked to a reduced risk of heart disease and stroke. They may also reduce inflammation and improve markers of diabetes

Downsides: Restricting fat too much can lead to health problems in the long term, as fat plays a key role in hormone production, nutrient absorption, and cell health. Moreover, very-low-fat diets have been linked to a higher risk of metabolic syndrome

Summary Low-fat diets restrict your intake of fat, as this macronutrient is higher in calories than protein and carbs. Studies have linked low-fat diets to weight loss and lower

risks of heart disease and diabetes.

6. The Mediterranean diet

The Mediterranean diet is based on foods that people in countries like Italy and Greece used to eat. Though it was designed to lower heart disease risk, numerous studies indicate that it can also aid in weight loss

How it works: The Mediterranean diet advocates eating plenty of fruits, vegetables, nuts, seeds, legumes, tubers, whole grains, fish, seafood, and extra virgin olive oil.

Foods such as poultry, eggs, and dairy products are to be eaten in moderation. Meanwhile, red meats are limited. Additionally, the Mediterranean diet restricts refined grains, trans fats, processed meats, added sugar, and other highly processed foods.

Weight loss: Though it's not specifically a weight loss diet, many studies show that adopting a Mediterranean-style diet may aid weight loss.

For example, an analysis of 19 studies found that people who combined the Mediterranean diet with exercise or calorie restriction lost an average of 8.8 pounds (4 kg) more than those on a control diet

Other benefits: The Mediterranean diet encourages eating plenty of antioxidant-rich foods, which may help combat inflammation and oxidative stress by neutralizing free radicals. It has been linked to reduced risks of heart disease and premature death

Downsides: As the Mediterranean diet is not strictly a weight loss diet, people may not lose weight following it unless they also consume fewer calories.

Summary The Mediterranean diet emphasizes eating plenty of fruits, vegetables, fish, and healthy oils while restricting refined and highly processed foods. While it's not a weight loss diet, studies show that it can promote weight loss and overall

health.

7. WW (Weight Watchers)

WW, formerly Weight Watchers, is one of the most popular weight loss programs worldwide. While it doesn't restrict any food groups, people on a WW plan must eat within their set daily points to reach their ideal weight

How it works: WW is a points-based system that assigns different foods and beverages a value, depending on their calorie, fat, and fiber contents. To reach your desired weight, you must stay within your daily point allowance.

Weight loss: Many studies show that the WW program can help you lose weight, For example, a review of 45 studies found that people who followed a WW diet lost 2.6% more weight than people who received standard counseling. What's more, people who follow WW programs are more successful at maintaining weight loss after several years, compared with those who follow other diets.

Other benefits: WW allows flexibility, making it easy to follow. This enables people with dietary restrictions, such as those with food allergies, to adhere to the plan.

Downsides: While it allows for flexibility, WW can be costly depending on the subscription plan. Also, its flexibility can be a downfall if dieters choose unhealthy foods.

Summary WW, or Weight Watchers, is a weight loss program that uses a points-based system. Studies show that it's effective for long-term weight loss and highly flexible.

8. The DASH diet

Dietary Approaches to Stop Hypertension, or DASH diet, is an eating plan that is designed to help treat or prevent high blood pressure, which is clinically known as hypertension.

It emphasizes eating plenty of fruits, vegetables, whole grains, and lean meats and is low in salt, red meat, added sugars, and fat. While the DASH diet is not a weight loss diet, many people report losing weight on it.

How it works: The DASH diet recommends specific servings of different food groups. The number of servings you are allowed to eat depends on your daily calorie intake.

For example, an average person on the DASH diet would eat about 5 servings of vegetables, 5 servings of fruit, 7 servings of healthy carbs like whole grains, 2 servings of low-fat dairy products, and 2 servings or fewer of lean meats per day. In addition, you're allowed to eat nuts and seeds 2–3 times per week

Weight loss: Studies show that the DASH diet can help you lose weight. For example, an analysis of 13 studies found that people on the DASH diet lost significantly more weight over 8–24 weeks than people on a control diet

Other benefits: The DASH diet has been shown to reduce blood pressure levels and several heart disease risk factors. Also, it may help combat recurrent depressive symptoms and lower your risk of breast and colorectal cancer

Downsides: While the DASH diet may aid weight loss, there is mixed evidence on salt intake and blood pressure. In addition, eating too little salt has been linked to increased insulin resistance and an increased risk of death in people with heart failure

Summary The DASH diet is a low-salt diet that has been shown to aid in weight loss. Studies have also linked it to additional benefits for your heart and reduced risks of other chronic diseases.

Many diets can help you lose weight. Some of the most well-researched diets and eating plans include intermittent fasting, plant-based diets, low-carb diets, low-fat diets, the paleo diet, the Mediterranean diet, WW (Weight Watchers), and the DASH diet.

While all of the above diets are effective for weight loss, the diet you choose should depend on your lifestyle and food preferences. This ensures that you are more likely to stick to it in the long term

CHAPTER TWO

Three Days Cardiac Diet as the Fastest And Easiest Weight Loss Plan

If the 3-day cardiac diet is one of the easiest and fastest ways to lose weight; so why haven't you heard of it? The odds are good that you have already heard of it, or at least something very much like the 3-day cardiac diet, which has also been called the Birmingham Hospital diet. This diet is one of a group of fairly similar diets that have been around for years, including the May Clinic Diet, the Grapefruit Diet, or the Cleveland Clinic diet.

The purpose of all these diets is to enable a person to lose as much weight as possible in three days. If you believe that the 3-day cardiac diet and diets like it came from these clinics, then the idea was to help cardiac patients lose the water weight and bloat before surgery. The institutions all deny that they originated these diets, but they are very effective at rapid weight loss. You will find the 3-day cardiac diet is a high protein, limited calorie diet that emphasizes vegetables and lean protein.

Because of the amounts of vegetables you're encouraged to eat, there's no risk of nutritional deficiencies arising, but you do need to make sure to only stay on it for three days at a time, or the low calories will cause a metabolic slowdown. For breakfast on each of the three days, you're going to want to focus on getting in protein as well as some fats, so the usual prescription is water-packed tuna or cottage cheese, about a half a cup's worth, and two eggs, cooked in your preferred style.

This gives you a good mix of protein and fat, which are important for maintaining your hunger at manageable levels and giving you the materials you need to keep your muscles strong. Under no circumstances should you skip breakfast or not eat the full amount. You may have coffee or tea with it, but make sure not to use sweeteners or any dairy products. Lunch will be a mixture of tuna and salad. On the first two days, you may have half a cup of water-packed tuna, and a salad of any size you like. Keep in mind, though, that the salad must be all vegetables – no cheese or croutons or the like... Make sure to use olive oil as your dressing, and don't skimp, you need good fats for proper metabolism.

On the third day of the 3-day cardiac diet, you may increase to a full cup. Dinner on the 3-day cardiac diet will consist of as much as you like of any kind of meat, prepared without sauce or breading. You need to back this up with two different types of vegetables, steamed and without sauce except for butter, which you should use on them. Do not eat bread, pasta, or potatoes on the 3-day cardiac diet, because it will disrupt the weight loss formula of the diet. Remember to drink at least 64 ounces of water while on the diet, and don't cheat, it's only three days. Follow these rules and the 3-day cardiac diet will give you quick and easy weight loss.

CHAPTER THREE

Three Day Diets a Fast Way To Lose Weight

There are a lot of three-day diets out there, and it's no surprise why they're so popular. The diets differ in what you get to eat and how you use them, but they all make the same promise: rapid weight loss. Very rapid weight loss. The general promise is six pounds throughout the diet. Since most people struggle to lose a pound a week, the promises of the three-day diets are very appealing. But these diets do raise two big questions; do they work and are they safe? Do they work? Yes and no. If you need to drop some pounds quickly to look your best for an event, then these three-day diets can be extremely effective, because if followed as instructed, they will help you drop pounds and inches.

The problem is that they aren't designed for long-term weight loss, which is why they are three-day diets and not thirty-year diets. They work mostly by causing a very rapid loss due to low carbohydrates and low salt content. This is fine because if you're using them as a quick fix, that's exactly what you want them to do. But the weight will come back almost immediately when you resume normal eating habits, which is true of pretty much every diet. The three-day diets are also, by their nature, very low in bulk, which means that your midsection will slim out quickly because there's not much in your intestines.

The three-day diets do lead to actual fat loss as well since by their nature they are low in calories and they are short enough that there is no metabolic slowdown as you would get if you stayed on the program longer. Depending on your size and activity level, it's unreasonable to expect to see from one to three pounds of actual fat loss. Are they safe? Yes, usually. Frankly, a lot of people worry about the safety of diets a lot more than they really should. The human body is an immensely adaptable machine, and you can eat pretty much anything foodwise for short periods with no ill effects, or anything at all.

Certainly, most of the three days diets are perfectly safe for a normal person who doesn't have a preexisting illness. You can't develop nutritional deficiencies over three days. In addition, most of the three-day diets have you eating healthier than the average person does normally. Typically, the diets have you eating mostly meat, vegetables, and fruit over the three days, and elimination starches and sugar. This is a big improvement over the way the normal person eats, and the chance of you becoming deficient in vitamins or nutrients, even over the long term, is virtually nonexistent. The problem with three-day diets is that they are also extremely low in calories, typically below 1000 calories, and often much below.

This is simply not enough calories even if you are trying to lose weight, and so you can't say that the three-day diets are safe for extended use. What you can do is do a three-on, four-off version of the diet. In the three days, do the diets exactly as planned, but for the next four days, eat the same foods without limiting portions. This will prevent metabolic slowdown and help make the three-day diets work for you.

CHAPTER FOUR

Lose Pounds In A Week With The Cabbage Soup Diet

If you want to lose pounds in a week, I recommend the Cabbage Soup diet. However, you should check with your Doctor or Health Professional first. This is a program where you can have unlimited bowls of cabbage soup, so you should never be hungry. Each day also brings a specific combination of foods to add variety to the diet. You should be able to shed 5 to 7 pounds when you lose pounds in a week with the Cabbage Soup Diet. As the base, you can either use chicken or beef bouillon to give it a meat flavor or V8 juice for more nutrition.

You'll want to make 48 ounces of broth for the following recipe. Saute 6 large green onions and then add them to the broth. Cut up 2 green peppers and add them. You will need one to two cans of tomatoes depending on your taste. Then chop and add 3 medium-sized carrots. 10 ounces of mushrooms is about the right amount. 1 bunch of celery chopped should be added. You will need to slice and put in at least half a head of cabbage (this is the Cabbage Soup diet after all).

Then you can season to taste with salt, pepper, parsley, curry, garlic powder, etc. Lose Pounds in a week by adding the following foods each day: Day 1: Eat any fruit you want except bananas. Do not substitute fruit juice. Day 2: Eat vegetables until you are stuffed. These can be raw or cooked. For dinner, you can add a big baked potato with butter. But don't eat fruit on this day. Day 3: All the fruits (except bananas) and vegetables (except potatoes) you want. Day 4: Up to 8 bananas and all the skim milk you want. This day is intended to reduce your desire for sweets. Day 5: This is an odd day for a diet. You must eat 6 tomatoes. Also, you can have 10 to 20 ounces of beef. Day 6: All the beef you want plus vegetables excluding potatoes. Day 7: (The final day).

Stuff yourself with brown rice, fruit juices, and vegetables. You should eat the soup at least once on this day, even if you are quite tired of it. How to lose pounds in a week on this diet is to follow the plan. The real trick may not be so much in the combination of foods but in the fact that you are unlikely to eat more than 1000 calories a day. However, if you deviate from the plan, you are likely to eat more than the 1000 calories, so stick to it. Also, you should know that it is impossible to be hungry on this diet so long as you eat the soup. You can have unlimited amounts of soup on this plan. It's not a good idea to do this diet indefinitely. If you want to continue with it, try a one-week on, one week off strategy. So, that's how to lose pounds in a week.

CHAPTER FIVE

Body Colon Cleanse Clear Your Intestines Lose Weight

The body colon cleanse is all the rage these days. What is it and why is so important to clean out a certain part of your intestines? You build up a lot of gunk in your system and this keeps you from losing weight. The body colon cleanse helps you lose weight by cleaning your system out. One body colon cleanse is called the lemonade diet. It was created by the late Naturopath Stanley Burroughs. It consists of fasting to rid the body of toxins, created by improper diet, lack of exercise, and negative mental attitudes.

The body colon cleanses will dissolve and eliminate toxins and congestion. It will cleanse the kidneys and digestive system. It aims to purify glands and eliminate waste and hardened materials in the joints and muscles. You'll start to build a healthy bloodstream which in turn leads to developing optimal blood pressure Also, the body colon cleanses will help you lose weight. Most people lose about 2 pounds a day with no harmful side effects.

The lemonade diet should be followed for exactly 10 days. During this period, you will not eat anything and you will only drink a specially formulated lemonade. You need to drink at least 10 servings of lemonade a day, which can be difficult to manage without discipline. The recipe for the lemonade is as follows: fill a one-gallon water jug with the juice of five lemons, 1 and ¼ cups of Organic Grade B maple syrup (no substitutes), 1/ 10 tsp. or more of cayenne pepper, and fill the rest of the jug with purified or spring water (do not use fluoridated tap water.) When you get up each morning that you are on the body colon cleanse, you need to do a salt water flush.

Mix two level teaspoons of unionized sea salt with a quart of lukewarm water and mix. Drink this all right away. Then in the evening, you'll want to take an herbal laxative tea which you can find in most grocery stores. You should be prepared to need to use the restroom a lot while on the body colon cleanse. Specifically, that means that you should be prepared to go every 15 or 20 minutes. If you have a job or other activities that will not accommodate this need, you may want to consider putting the program off until you can use the facilities whenever you need to. You may think that drinking only lemonade, saltwater, and tea with no food for 10 days is dangerous. Well, you are certainly not going to die on this diet, but you will be hungry.

Surprisingly, you will probably find that you have more energy as the diet goes on, despite the lack of food. At the end of the body, colon cleanses, you can expect to have lost anywhere from 5 to 10 pounds (this is mostly water weight and will be quickly regained if you don't follow a reasonable eating and exercise plan), feel increased energy, have an increased desire to eat healthy foods, and feel somewhat different about life in general. Those who make it through a body colon cleanse are generally very glad that they did it.

CHAPTER SIX

Eat Out To Lose Weight With A Restaurant Calorie Counter

A restaurant calorie counter can be a dieter's best friend. Losing weight isn't easy, so you need to take steps to make it as easy as possible on yourself. One way to do this is to not limit yourself to just bland home meals and a life where you never eat out for fear of not being able to maintain your diet the way you want to. With a restaurant calorie counter, you won't have to. There's no doubt that losing weight is difficult.

The rate of obesity is soaring and it's not because people are trying to gain weight, sumo wrestlers excepted. In general, more than 95 percent of people who do manage to lose weight won't be able to keep it off. Many people manage to gain and lose hundreds of pounds over their lifetime. When something is this difficult, you need to take every step you can to make it as easy as possible. This includes eating out or grabbing things on the fly, which is where a restaurant calorie counter comes in handy.

We'd all like to be able to do up our food at home, eat perfectly all day and come back to prepare a nutritionally flawless means for dinner, all with a smile on our face. But in reality, this doesn't happen. People sleep late, work late, and sometimes the boss wants you to have lunch with him. It's a rare person who can get by without buying their food already prepared at some point.

Unless your eating out is going to consist of glasses of water, you're going to need a restaurant calorie counter. A restaurant calorie counter is pretty much exactly what it sounds like. It's a guide to the calories and nutrient contents of things you find in restaurants. Generally, these will be available for all chain-type restaurants, fast food, and otherwise, but a very good restaurant calorie counter will also have very famous restaurants, and it is possible to get copies that have local information, as well. The local restaurants are a flaw in using a restaurant calorie counter; even those that have restaurants are forced to estimate.

This isn't necessarily a huge problem but bears in mind that if you're eating at Uncle Joe's Wings and Things you're going to have to estimate. A good way to do this, if you're eating in a place where you're going to be eating a lot but the place isn't listed in your restaurant calorie counter, is to get your favorites as taking out. Once you have them, measure them and then find something on the counter that's pretty close and work out how many calories are in each one. Either way, a restaurant calorie counter can be key to your weight loss success, regardless of the type of diet you're on. If you're using a controlled calorie plan, then you can easily look up the calorie count and adjust. Or you can choose dishes with the right amount of fat or carbs for your plan. Every diet is easier with a restaurant calorie counter.

CHAPTER SEVEN

Diet Slimming Pills Which Ones Are Good

Diet Slimming Pills Which Ones Are Good Diet slimming pills abound on the market. Which ones are good and which ones should you forgo? And, how can you tell if something is a scam? This article will explore the real world of diet slimming pills. Diet slimming pills are not tested or regulated by the federal government if they are sold as supplements and not medicines. If you don't have to get it for a pharmacist, it is not FDA approved. But it's not FDA disproved either. This applies to supplements bought at a local drug store and ones bought over the internet.

Every six months or so, the media picks up on a new natural substance that seems to help with weight loss. A few years back, that was Hoodia. More recently it was Acai Berry. Hoodia makes for a very interesting case study. Bushmen in South Africa use a specific kind of hoodia and it makes them be able to live without food and with limited water for several days. However, there are about 20 other kinds of hoodia.

The hoodia that the Bushmen use is not available for marketing in the west because there are very limited quantities. South Africa is working on mass cultivation for weight loss purposes, but at this point, it is not in any diet slimming pills. That said, there are no limits on the number of supplements claiming they have the "correct" hoodia in them. Many people who use these diet slimming pills are disappointed to find that they do not curb the appetite at all.

A more recent case study is the Acai Berry. Many companies are advertising that Rachael Ray and Oprah have endorsed Acai Berry. While both have run segments on the nutritional benefits of the actual fruit, they have not endorsed any of these diet slimming pills. The supplements which claim to be Ray and Oprah endorsed often have only minute traces of the fruit in them and certainly not enough to have any real dieting help. They do, however, have a lot of caffeine in them which can be harmful to some people. Hoodia, Acai Berry, and other kinds of supplement products are notorious for poor customer service.

The Tuscon Better Business Bureau has received more than 150 complaints against just one company that sells Acai Berry, most related to billing. One thing to watch for with these diet slimming pills is free trial offers. This is a bait and switch. Usually, the trial starts the day you order the product, not the day you receive it. You may receive your pills on day 12 of a 14-day trial offer. If you don't ship them back immediately, you will be billed the full amount.

It is generally better to bite the bullet and fork out the entire amount upfront if a supplement looks like it might be a good thing rather than sign up for a continuity program that has a free trial period. Ultimately, you have to decide whether a diet slimming product is right for you. Just don't believe everything you see in advertising.

CHAPTER EIGHT

Ketosis Diet Low Carb Programs

Do you want to go on a Ketosis diet? Several popular diet plans are based on this principle. Adkins and South Beach are both diets that restrict carbs. This results in a ketosis diet. The theory behind a ketosis diet is that your body will burn fat rather than carbohydrates if you deprive it of almost all carbohydrate sources. This means limiting your carb intake to just 20 grams in some cases.

Normally, the carbohydrates in food are converted into glucose. The glucose is then transported through the body and is particularly important in fuelling the brain. However, if there are very few carbs in the diet, the liver converts fat into fatty acids and ketone bodies. The ketone bodies pass into the brain and replace glucose as an energy source. Thus, the body produces ketone bodies—a state known as ketosis.

Low Carb diets take advantage of this state of ketosis. Since cells in the body can use ketones for energy instead of glucose, and since ketones are easier to produce, only a small amount of glucose is created. In other words, ketosis is the more significant process in this case. Diets low in starches and sugars do not directly affect blood sugar levels significantly, meals tend to have a little direct effect on insulin levels. These diets tend to discourage insulin production in general.

Additionally, many experts argue that a ketosis diet is more like the diet our bodies have evolved to use. Before the advent of agriculture just a few thousand years ago, the human body had millions of years of evolution which were selected for a hunter gathered lifestyle. Hunter-gatherers had very few carbs in their diets. They may have had the original ketosis diet.

Dr. Robert Adkins first published the Adkins Diet Revolution in 1972 which set off the modern round of low-carb dieting. At the time, its appeal was limited because so many scientists and doctors condemned it. Over time, though, it gained credibility and when he republished the book as Dr. Adkins's New Diet Revolution, it set off a frenzy.

Soon other ketosis diet books appeared. These included the popular South Beach diet, Zone diet, and Protein Power. While the scientific community still hasn't acknowledged the value of the ketosis diet, they have started to make recommendations that people reduce the number of carbohydrates in their diets. The medical community has stressed the importance of fiber in diets and recommended that children not drink juice regularly.

While the popularity of ketosis diets has waned since its height in 2004, there are still many adherents. That's because, for many people, low-carb diets work when nothing else has before.

There has been much scientific research on low-carb diets. Many studies show it works and many studies show that it is dangerous. Because of these competing studies, advocates on both sides can pull up evidence that they are right. Once you do your due diligence, you will be better able to decide whether to pursue a ketosis diet.

CHAPTER NINE

How to Lose Weight Fast: 3 Simple Steps, Based on Science.

If your doctor recommends it, there are ways to lose weight safely. A steady weight loss of 1 to 2 pounds per week is recommended for the most effective long-term weight management. hat said many eating plans leave you feeling hungry or unsatisfied. These are major reasons why you might find it hard to stick to a healthier eating plan. However, not all diets have this effect. Low carb diets and whole-food, lower-calorie diets are effective for weight loss and may be easier to stick to than other diets.

Here are some ways to lose weight that employ healthy eating, potentially lower carbs, and that aim to:

- reduce your appetite
- cause fast weight loss
- improve your metabolic health at the same time

How to Lose Weight Fast in 3 Simple Steps

1. Cut back on refined carbs

One way to lose weight quickly is to cut back on sugars and starches, or carbohydrates. This could be with a low-carb eating plan or by reducing refined carbs and replacing them with whole grains. When you do that, your hunger levels go down, and you generally end up eating fewer calories With a low-carb eating plan, you'll utilize burning stored fat for energy instead of carbs.

If you choose to eat more complex carbs like whole grains along with a calorie deficit, you'll benefit from higher fiber and digest them more slowly.

This makes them more filling to keep you satisfied. A 2020 study confirmed that a very low carbohydrate diet was beneficial for losing weight in older populations Research also suggests that a low carb diet can reduce appetite, which may lead to eating fewer calories without thinking about it or feeling hungry

Note that the long-term effects of a low-carb diet are still being researched. It can also be difficult to adhere to a low-carb diet, which may lead to yo-yo dieting and less success in maintaining a healthy weight. There are potential downsides to a low-carb diet that may lead you to a different method. Reduced calorie diets can also lead to weight loss and be easier to maintain for longer periods.

If you opt for a diet focusing instead on whole grains over refined carbs, a 2019 study correlated high whole grain with lower body mass index (BMI) To determine the best way for you to lose weight, consult your doctor for recommendations.

SUMMARY

Reducing sugars and starches, or carbs, from your diet can help curb your appetite, lower your insulin levels, and make you lose weight. But the long-term effects of a low-carb diet are not yet known. A reduced-calorie diet could be more sustainable.

2. Eat protein, fat, and vegetables

Each one of your meals should include:

- a protein source
- fat source
- vegetables
- a small portion of complex carbohydrates, such as whole grains

To see how you can assemble your meals, check out:

- this low carb meal plan
- this lower calorie meal plan
- these lists of 101 healthy low carb recipes and low-calorie foods

Protein

Eating a recommended amount of protein is essential to help preserve your health and muscle mass while losing weight Evidence suggests that eating adequate protein may improve cardiometabolic risk factors, appetite, and body weight,

Here's how to determine how much you need to eat without eating too much. Many factors determine your specific needs, but generally, an average person needs (9Trusted Source):

- 56–91 grams per day for the average male
- 46–75 grams per day for the average female

Diets with adequate protein can also help:

- reduce cravings and obsessive thoughts about food by 60%
- reduce the desire to snack late at night by half
- make you feel full

In one study, people on a higher protein diet ate 441 fewer calories per day.

Healthy protein sources include:

- **meat:** beef, chicken, pork, and lamb
- **fish and seafood:** salmon, trout, and shrimp
- **eggs:** whole eggs with the yolk
- **plant-based proteins:** beans, legumes, quinoa, tempeh, and tofu

Low carb and leafy green vegetables

Don't be afraid to load your plate with leafy green vegetables. They're packed with nutrients, and you can eat very large amounts without greatly increasing calories and carbs.

Vegetables to include for low carb or low-calorie eating plans:

- broccoli
- cauliflower
- spinach
- tomatoes
- kale
- Brussels sprouts
- cabbage
- Swiss chard
- lettuce

- cucumber

Healthy fats

Don't be afraid of eating fats.

Your body still requires healthy fats no matter what eating plan you choose. Olive oil and avocado oil are great choices for including in your eating plan.

Other fats such as butter and coconut oil should be used only in moderation due to their higher saturated fat content (12Trusted Source).

SUMMARY

Assemble each meal out of a protein source, healthy fat source, complex carb, and vegetables. Leafy green vegetables are a great way to bulk up a meal with low calories and lots of nutrients.

3. Move your body

Exercise, while not required to lose weight, can help you lose weight more quickly. Lifting weights has particularly good benefits. By lifting weights, you'll burn lots of calories and prevent your metabolism from slowing down, which is a common side effect of losing weight

Try going to the gym three to four times a week to lift weights. If you're new to the gym, ask a trainer for some advice. Make sure your doctor is also aware of any new exercise plans. If lifting weights is not an option for you, doing some cardio workouts such as walking, jogging, running, cycling, or swimming is very beneficial for weight loss and general health.

Both cardio and weightlifting can help with weight loss.

SUMMARY

Resistance training, such as weightlifting, is a great option for losing weight. If that's not possible, cardio workouts are also effective. Choose what's sustainable for you.

What about calories and portion control?

If you opt for a low-carb eating plan, it's not necessary to count calories as long as you keep your carb intake very low and stick to protein, fat, and low-carb vegetables. If you find yourself not losing weight, you may want to keep track of your calories to see if that's a contributing factor. If you're sticking to a calorie deficit to lose weight, you can use a free online calculator like this one.

Enter your sex, weight, height, and activity levels. The calculator will tell you how many calories to eat per day to maintain your weight, lose weight, or lose weight fast. You can also download free, easy-to-use calorie counters from websites and app stores. Here's a list of 5 calorie counters to try. Note that eating too few calories can be dangerous and less effective for losing weight. Aim to reduce your calories by a sustainable and healthy amount based on your doctor's recommendation.

SUMMARY

Counting calories isn't usually needed to lose weight on a low-carb eating plan. But if you're not losing weight or on a reduced-calorie eating plan, calorie counting may help.

9 weight loss tips

Here are 9 more tips to lose weight faster:

1. **Eat a high-protein breakfast.** Eating a high-protein breakfast could help reduce cravings and calorie intake throughout the day.
2. **Avoid sugary drinks and fruit juice.** Empty calories from sugar aren't useful to your body and can hinder weight loss
3. **Drink water before meals.** One study showed that drinking water before meals reduced calorie intake and may be effective in weight management
4. **Choose weight-loss-friendly foods.** Some foods are better for weight loss than others. Here is a list of healthy weight-loss-friendly foods.
5. **Eat soluble fiber.** Studies show that soluble fibers may promote weight loss. Fiber supplements like glucomannan can also help
6. **Drink coffee or tea.** Caffeine consumption can boost your metabolism
7. **Base your diet on whole foods.** They're healthier, more filling, and much less likely to cause overeating than processed foods.
8. **Eat slowly.** Eating quickly can lead to weight gain over time while eating slowly makes you feel more full and boosts weight-reducing hormones
9. **Get good quality sleep.** Sleep is important for many reasons, and poor sleep is one of the biggest risk factors for weight gain

For more tips on weight loss, read about natural tips for losing weight here.

SUMMARY

Eating whole foods, higher protein, soluble fiber, and less sugar can help you lose more weight. Don't forget to get a good night's sleep, too.

Sample meal ideas for fast weight loss

These sample meal plans are low carb, which limits carbs to 20–50 carbs per day. Each meal should have protein, healthy fats, and veggies.

If you'd prefer to lose weight while still eating complex carbs, add in some healthy whole grains such as:

- quinoa
- whole oats
- whole wheat
- bran
- rye
- barley

Breakfast ideas

- poached egg with sliced avocado and a side of berries
- spinach, mushroom, and feta crustless quiche
- green smoothie with spinach, avocado, and nut milk and a side of cottage cheese
- unsweetened Greek yogurt with berries and almonds

Lunch ideas

- smoked salmon with avocado and a side of asparagus
- lettuce wrap with grilled chicken, black beans, red pepper, and salsa
- kale and spinach salad with grilled tofu, chickpeas, and guacamole
- BLT wrap with celery sticks and peanut butter

Dinner ideas

- enchilada salad with chicken, peppers, mango, avocado, and spices
- ground turkey bake with mushrooms, onions, peppers, and cheese
- antipasto salad with white beans, asparagus, cucumbers, olive oil, and Parmesan
- roasted cauliflower with tempeh, Brussels sprouts, and pine nuts
- salmon baked with ginger, sesame oil, and roasted zucchini

Snack ideas

- cauliflower hummus and veggies
- healthy homemade trail mix with nuts and dried fruit

- kale chips
- cottage cheese with cinnamon and flaxseeds
- spicy roasted chickpeas
- roasted pumpkin seeds
- tuna pouches
- steamed edamame
- strawberries and brie

How fast will you lose weight?

You may lose 5–10 pounds (2.3–4.5 kg) of weight — sometimes more — in the first week of a diet plan and then lose weight consistently after that. The first week is usually a loss of both body fat and water weight.

If you're new to dieting, weight loss may happen more quickly. The more weight you have to lose, the faster you'll lose it. Unless your doctor suggests otherwise, losing 1–2 pounds per week is usually a safe amount. If you're trying to lose weight faster than that, speak to your doctor about a safe level of calorie reduction.

Aside from weight loss, a low carb diet can improve your health in a few ways, though the long-term effects are not yet known:

- blood sugar levels tend to significantly decrease on low carb diets (30)
- triglycerides tend to go down (31)
- LDL (bad) cholesterol goes down (32Trusted Source)
- blood pressure improves significantly (33Trusted Source)

Other diet types that reduce calories and increase whole foods are also associated with improved metabolic markers and slower aging (34, 35Trusted Source, 36Trusted Source). Ultimately, you may find a more balanced diet that includes complex carbohydrates is more sustainable.

SUMMARY

Significant weight can be lost on a low carb or low-calorie diet, but the speed depends on the individual. General weight loss can improve certain markers of health, such as blood sugar and cholesterol levels.

The Bottom Line

By reducing carbs or replacing refined carbs with complex carbs, you'll likely experience reduced appetite and hunger. This removes the main reasons it's often difficult to maintain a weight loss plan.

With a sustainable low carb or lower-calorie eating plan, you can eat healthy food until you're full and still lose a significant amount of fat.

The initial drop in water weight can lead to a drop in the scales within a few days. Fat loss takes longer

Printed by Libri Plureos GmbH in Hamburg,
Germany